Low Carb Dieting
101

21 Mouth Watering Recipes for the Low Card Dieter

Table of Contents

Introduction

Conclusion

Introduction

Eating healthy and losing weight is hard and often confusing. This complete low-carb cookbook includes a great collection of low carb recipes. The delicious and healthy recipes of this cookbook taste so good you will forget that you are on a diet. Several scientific studies show that people who follow a low-carb diet lose weight faster than any other diets. Time and time again, scientists have been telling us that "It's not fat, but carbohydrates that make us fat."

Scientists and health experts agree that we should eat fewer carbohydrates to lose weight and live longer. Dieting doesn't have to be about sacrificing or feeling bored. Having enough variety and choices to keep the dieter from losing interest is one of the toughest challenges of any diet. Dieters will be pleased to know that with low carb diet, they can eat foods like sausage, pizza, quiche, casserole and dessert without giving up great taste and still lose weight. With this collection of low carb recipes, you will feel fuller, healthy and satisfied.

Chapter 1
Breakfast Recipes

Blueberry Muffins

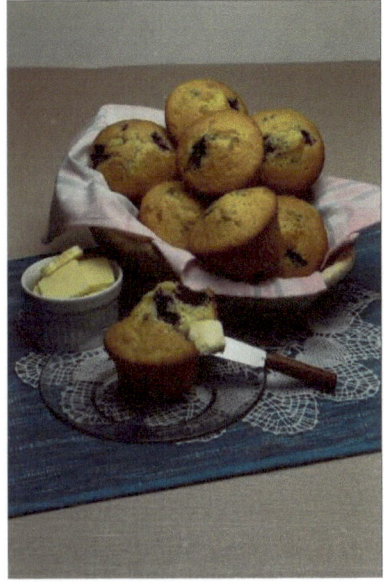

Ingredients for 15 muffins

- o   Almond flour – 2 cups

- o   Heavy cream – 1 cup

- o   Eggs - 2

- o   Melted butter – 1/8 cup

- o   Artificial sweetener such as stevia or Splenda – 5 packets

- o   Baking soda – ½ teaspoon

- o   Lemon extract or flavoring – ½ teaspoon

- o   Dried lemon zest – ½ teaspoon

- o   Salt – ¼ teaspoon

- o   Fresh blueberries – 4 ounces

Method

1. Preheat the oven to 350F. This recipe makes 15 muffins, so place cupcake papers in individual muffin holes of two regular sized 12 count muffin pans.

2. Mix cream and almond flour in a bowl.

3. One at a time, mix eggs and stir until mixed.

4. Add baking soda, sweetener, butter, spices and flavoring and mix.

5. Now add blueberries and stir to distribute evenly.

6. Fill each cupcake cup about ½ full with batter.

7. Bake until golden, about 20 minutes.

8. Let cool and serve with butter.

Nutrition Facts Per Serving

- Calories 184
- Carb 6 g
- Protein 5 g
- Fiber 2 g
- Fat 17 g

Low Carb Quiche

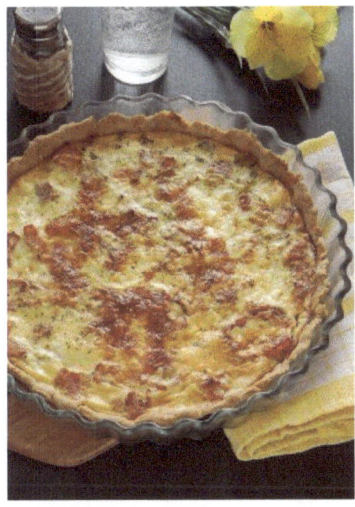

Ingredients for 2 quiches

- ○ Colby jack and or shredded muenster cheese divided in half

- ○ Butter – 2 tablespoons, plus more for greasing pans

- ○ White onion – 1 large, finely chopped

- ○ Organic eggs – 12 large

- ○ Heavy cream – 2 cups

- ○ Salt – 1 teaspoon

- ○ Ground black pepper – 1 teaspoon

- ○ Dried thyme – 2 teaspoons

Method

1. Preheat the oven to 350F.

2. Melt the butter in a separated skillet over medium-low heat. Add the vegetables and sauté until onions are soft and translucent. Remove the vegetables from heat and cool.

3. Butter two deep pie pans or 10-inch quiche pans. In the bottom of each buttered pan, put 2 cups of shredded cheese. To each pan, add ½ of cooled vegetable mixture in an even layer over cheese.

4. Into a large mixing bowl, crack 12 eggs. Add the spices and cream and whisk together until the mixture is well mixed and frothy. Over each pan of vegetables and cheese, pour ½ mixture. Then with a fork, gently and evenly distribute vegetables and cheese into egg-cream mixture.

5. Place the quiche pans into the oven. Make sure there is an inch of space between pans. Bake until set and puffy, and the center is slightly golden, about 20-25 minutes. The quiches are done when a knife inserted into the middle comes out clean.

6. Cut the quiches and serve.

Nutrition Facts Per Serving

- Calories 382
- Protein 16 g
- Fat 33 g
- Carb 5 g
- Fiber 1 g

Egg, Turkey, and Spinach Muffin Cups

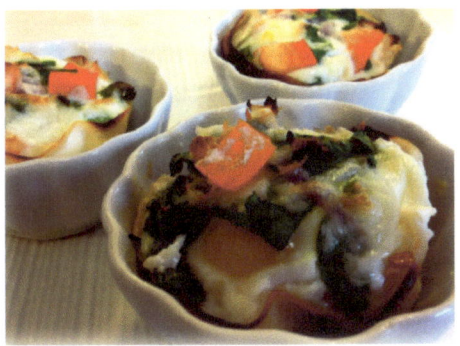

Ingredients for 6 muffin cups

- o Salt and pepper to taste
- o Red onion – 2 tablespoons, finely chopped
- o Fresh basil as needed
- o Mozzarella Cheese Light as needed
- o Eggs – 6
- o Nitrate Free Shaved Turkey – 6 slices
- o Spinach – ½ cup, sliced
- o Red pepper – 3 tablespoons

Method

1. Preheat the oven to 350F.

2. Grate the mozzarella cheese and slice the red onion, red pepper, spinach, and basil.

3. Spray a nonstick muffin tin with olive oil spray.

4. Place the turkey slices first in the muffin cups, so that they rest on the bottom and the sides of the tin to make a larger cup.

5. Into each of the turkey cup, carefully crack an egg.

6. Add a little bit of sliced red pepper, spinach, red onion, and cheese on top of the egg.

7. Sprinkle some fresh basil onto the eggs, and season with salt and pepper.

8. Place the muffin tin in the oven and bake. It takes about 10 minutes for a runny yolk and about 15 minutes for a harder one. Also, remember, that the egg muffins will continue to cook when you take it out of the oven.

9. Cool and serve.

Nutrition Facts Per Serving

- Calories 95
- Protein 9 g
- Fat 6 g
- Carb 2 g

Egg White Spinach Omelet

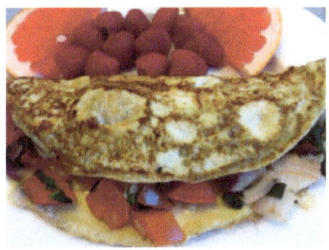

Ingredients

- Egg whites – 4 or 5
- Egg yolk – 1
- Almond milk or coconut milk – 2 tablespoons (30 ml)
- Plum tomato – 1
- Shredded spinach – 1 handful
- Purple onion – 1 tablespoon
- Basil – 1 pinch
- Garlic as needed
- Olive oil cooking spray

Method

1. Chop the vegetables and beat the almond milk, egg whites, and yolk.

2. Spray a frying pan with oil and then sauté the vegetables until just soft.

3. Place the vegetables on the side. Then spray the pan again. Place on medium-low heat and pour the eggs.

4. Cook until the eggs are firm. Now add the vegetables on one side and fold the other half over top.

5. Add fruits to the plate and serve

Egg Scramble

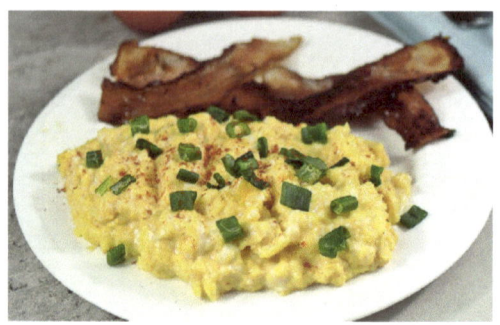

Ingredients for 2 servings

- Eggs – 2
- Butter – 2 tablespoons
- Sour cream – 2 tablespoons
- Green onion – 2 stalks
- Bacon – 4 strips
- Salt – ½ teaspoon
- Garlic powder – ½ teaspoon
- Onion powder – ½ teaspoon
- Black powder – ¼ teaspoon
- Paprika – ¼ teaspoon

Method

1. Into a cold, ungreased pan, crack the eggs and add the butter. (Once they are on the heat, start mixing the eggs. Season the eggs only when they are cooked.)

2. Place the pan over medium-high heat and with a silicone spatula, begin stirring the butter and eggs.

3. While stirring the eggs, bake or cook some bacon strips.

4. Alternate stirring the eggs on and off the heat and never stop stirring the eggs.

5. Slowly, the eggs should start coming together. Turn the heat off when the eggs are almost cooked. The eggs will continue to cook from the residual heat from the pan.

6. Add 2 tablespoons of sour cream and season with paprika, pepper, onion powder, garlic powder, and salt.

7. Now add two stalks of chopped green onion.

8. Add the bacon when the eggs are cooked.

9. Serve.

Nutrition Facts Per Serving

- Calories 444
- Fat 35 g
- Protein 25 g
- Carb 2 g

Chapter 2
Lunch
Recipes

Danish Meatballs

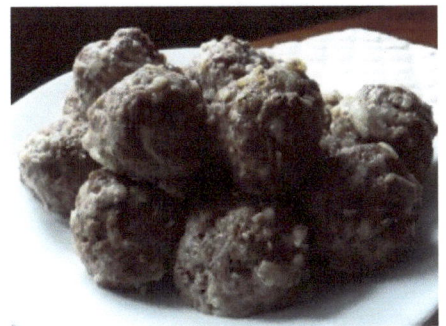

Ingredients for 30-1 ounce portions

- o   White onion – 4 ounces, minced

- o   Butter – 1 tablespoon

- o   Swiss cheese – 4 ounces

- o   Cold whole milk ricotta cheese – 1 cup

- o   Cold egg – 1 large

- o   Nutmeg – 1.5 teaspoons

- o   Allspice – 1.5 teaspoons

- o   Sea salt – 1,5 teaspoons

- o   Freshly ground black pepper – ½ teaspoon

- o   Ground beef – 1 pound (92% lean)

Method

1. In a skillet, sauté onions in butter until translucent. Remove from heat and cool for 10-12 minutes.

2. Meanwhile, shred the Swiss cheese. Then in a food processor, mince the shreds to a fine crumble. Set aside.

3. Combine egg and ricotta cheese in a mixing bowl and whisk.

4. Add the spices, and season with salt and pepper, mix well.

5. Add Swiss cheese and onions and mix until smooth.

6. Now add the beef to the mixture and mix until all ingredients are combined and become a non-sticky "dough"

7. Divide meat mixture into 30-1 ounce sized pieces. Then roll each piece into a ball.

8. Place the meatballs on a cookie sheet, and bake at 350F for 20 minutes, or until cooked through and brown.

Nutrition Facts Per Serving

- Calories 62
- Fat 4 g
- Protein 5 g
- Carb 1 g

Cobb Salad

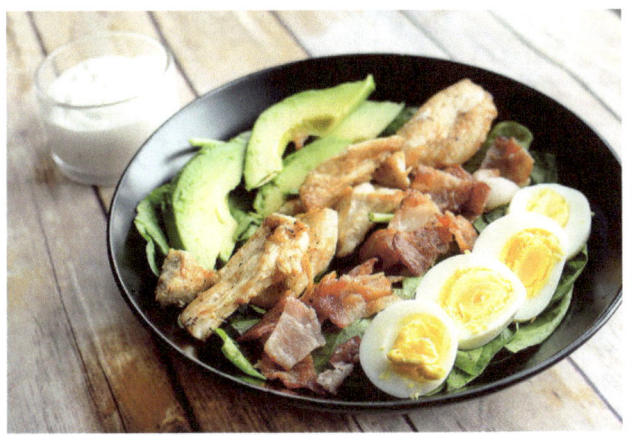

Ingredients for 1 serving

- o   Spinach – 1 cup

- o   Hard-boiled egg – 1

- o   Bacon – 2 strips

- o   Chicken breast – 2 oz.

- o   Campari tomato – ½

- o   Avocado – ¼

- o   White vinegar – ½ teaspoon

- o   Olive oil – 1 tablespoon

Method

1. Cook your bacon and chicken. Slice or shred your chicken.

2. Chop up all the ingredients into bite-sized pieces.

3. In a large mixing bowl, combine them with oil and vinegar.

4. Toss well and enjoy.

Nutrition Facts Per Serving

- Calories 600
- Protein 43 g
- Fat 48 g
- Carb 3 g

Tomato Soup

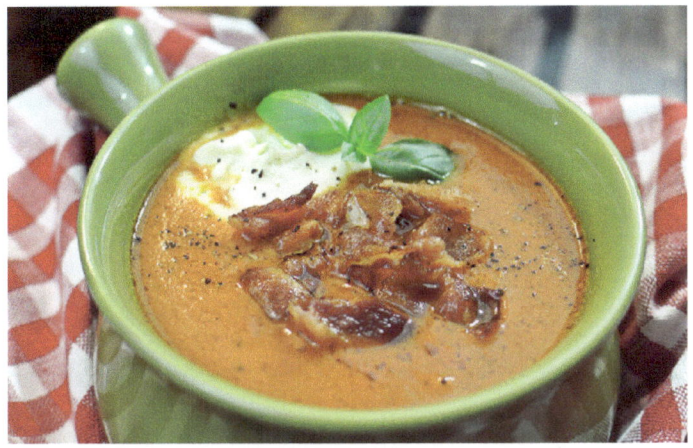

Ingredients for 4 servings

Main ingredients

- o   Tomato soup – 1 quart
- o   Olive oil – ¼ cup
- o   Butter – 4 tablespoons
- o   Frank's RedHot Sauce – ¼ cup
- o   Apple cider vinegar – 2 tablespoons

Spices

- o   Pink Himalayan sea salt – 1 tablespoon
- o   Black pepper – 2 teaspoons
- o   Oregano – 1 teaspoon
- o   Turmeric – 2 teaspoons

Toppings

- Fresh basil

- Green onion

- Cream Fraiche – 4 tablespoons

- Bacon – 8 strips

Method

1. In a pan, cook your bacon to a crisp while you prepare your tomato soup.

2. In a pot, combine all the main ingredients and place on a medium heat and stir.

3. Add the spices and cook until the butter is melted. Careful not to boil the soup, just a simmer is needed.

4. Pour the soup into soup bowls. Top with crème Fraiche, basil, some green onion and crispy bacon.

Nutrition Facts Per Serving

- Calories 460
- Protein 11 g
- Fat 37.5 g
- Carb 16 g

Shrimp with Garlic Sauce

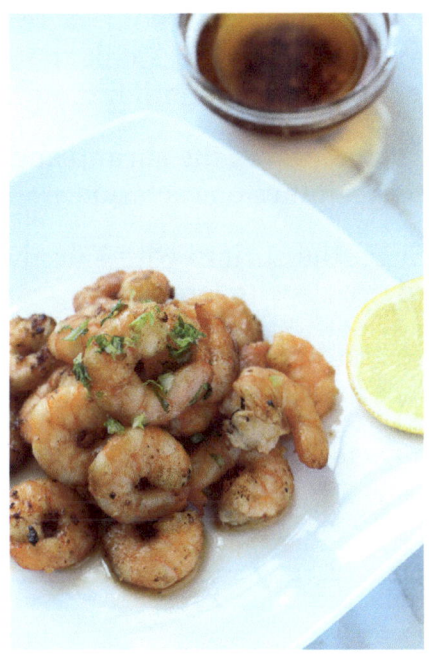

Ingredients for 2 servings

- o   Large shrimp – ½ lb
- o   Olive oil – ¼ cup
- o   Garlic – 3 cloves, minced
- o   Cayenne – ¼ teaspoon
- o   Lemon – 1 wedge
- o   Salt and pepper to taste

Method

1. Into a small pan, pour olive oil with cayenne and garlic. Cook the garlic on medium-low heat until fragrant.

2. Peel and devein the shrimp and cook for 2 to 3 minutes on each side.

3. Season the shrimp with salt and pepper and drizzle with lemon juice.

4. Use the leftover garlic oil as a dipping sauce and serve.

Nutrition Facts Per Serving

- Calories 335
- Protein 22.3 g
- Fat 27 g
- Carb 2.5 g

Fish Tacos

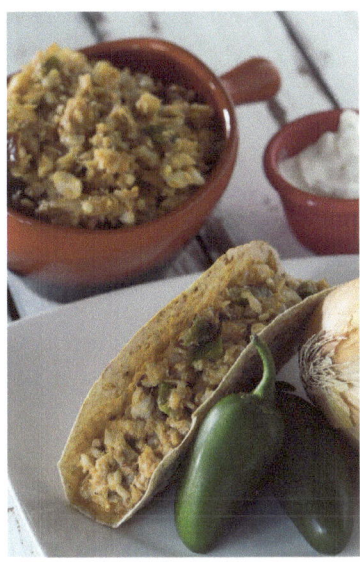

Ingredients for 4 servings

- o   Olive oil – 2 tablespoons

- o   Small yellow onion – 1/2, diced

- o   Fresh jalapeno – 1, chopped

- o   Garlic – 2 cloves, pressed

- o   Chipotle peppers in adobo sauce – 4 oz.

- o   Butter – 2 tablespoons

- o   Mayonnaise – 2 tablespoons

- o   Haddock fillets – 1 lb

- o   Low carb tortillas – 4

Method

1. Heat olive oil in a tall pan over medium-high heat. Then fry the diced onion for 5 minutes, or until translucent.

2. Lower the heat to medium, add the garlic and jalapeno and cook for another 2 minutes, stir continuously.

3. Add the adobe sauce and chopped chipotles to the pan.

4. Add the fish fillets, mayo and butter to the pan.

5. Mix everything until the fish is fully cooked, about 8 minutes.

6. Now fry the tortilla in a pan (2 minutes per side) on high heat.

7. Allow to cool the tortillas and fill them with the fish mix.

Nutrition Facts Per Serving

- Calories 300
- Fat 20 g
- Protein 24 g
- Carb 7 g

Cauliflower Salmon

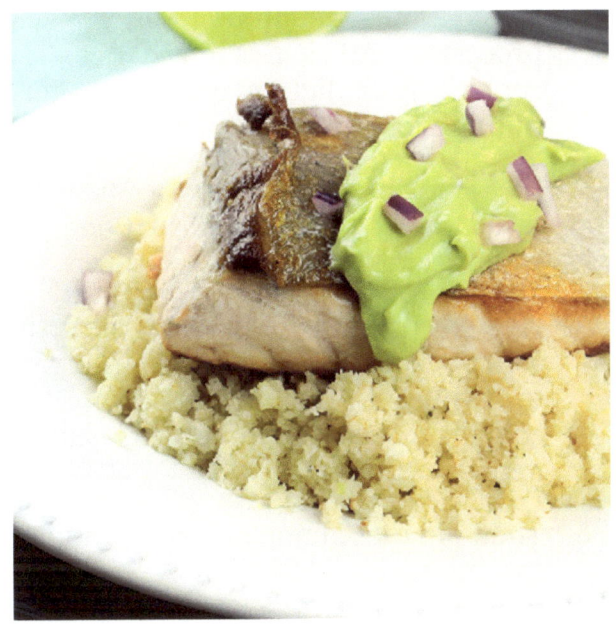

Ingredients for 2 servings

- o   Salmon fillets – 26 oz.

- o   Avocado – 1

- o   Lime – ½

- o   Red onion – 2 tablespoons, diced

- o   Cauliflower – 100 grams

Method

1. Pulse your cauliflower in a food processor until it resembled rice. Then cook it in a lightly oiled pan, for 8 minutes, covered.

2. Blend together the juice of ½ a lime, diced the red onion and avocado until smooth and creamy.

3. Heat a skillet over medium heat, add some oil and cook the salmon fillet for 4 to 5 minutes, skin side down. While cooking, season the fillet with salt and pepper.

4. Then flip the salmon and cook another 4 to 5 minutes.

5. Remove from heat when cooked. Spread the cauliflower rice over a serving plate. Top with the salmon and a generous dollop of your avocado lime sauce.

Nutrition Facts Per Serving

- Calories 420
- Fat 27 g
- Protein 37 g
- Carb 5 g

Low Carb Pizza

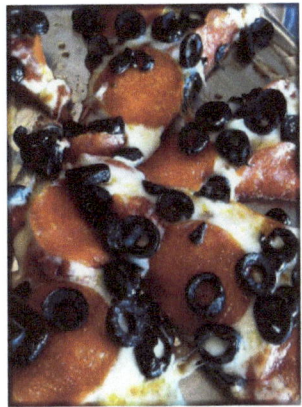

Ingredients for 1 pizza

- Olive oil – 1 tablespoon

- Organic cauliflower – 1 large head, trimmed and chopped into small pieces

- White onion – 1.5 ounces, minced

- Butter – 2 tablespoons

- Water – ¼ cup

- Low-carb pizza sauce – 1 (14 ounce) jar

- Low-carb Italian sausage – 1 pound

- Eggs – 3

- Shredded mozzarella cheese – 2 cups, chopped into smaller bits in a food processor.

- Fennel seed – 1 teaspoon

- Italian seasoning – 2 teaspoons

- Grated Parmesan – ¼ cup

- Shredded Italian 5 cheese blend – 2 cups

For the crust

- Preheat the oven to 450F. Then grease a 17 X 11 cookie sheet with olive oil.

- Melt the butter in a large skillet with a lid. Then add the cauliflower and onion. Over low to medium heat, sauté the vegetables until the cauliflower is almost done.

- Add the water, cover the skillet and steam the cauliflower until completely soft. Remove from heat, transfer to a ceramic or glass bowl to cool.

- Meanwhile, add the Italian sausage to the skillet and cook. With a spatula, break it up into smaller pieces. Cook until done. Remove the sausage from the skillet and place in a bowl, cover with paper towels to remove excess fat. Set aside to cool.

- Measure out 3 cups of cooled cauliflower and place in a food processor. Process until it reaches a smooth consistency. Scrap the pureed cauliflower into a bowl.

- Add the Parmesan cheese, spices minced mozzarella cheese and eggs to the cauliflower. Mix well.

- Spread the cauliflower mixture on the greased cookie sheet with a spatula. Make the spread an even thickness.

- At 450F, bake the crust until the surface looks cooked and brown around edges, about 20 minutes.

- Meanwhile, chop up the cooked sausage into finer pieces.

- In a small saucepan, pour the sauce from the jar. Then add the chopped Italian sausage. Cover the saucepan, then over low to medium heat, bring to a slow simmer.

- Remove the crust from the oven when it is done. Then switch oven setting to broil. Place oven shelf about 4 inches from broiler.

- Pour the sausage and sauce mixture over the top of the crust, then with a spatula, spread the mixture. The coating will be very thin.

- With the Italian cheese blend, cover the crust and sauce evenly.

- Place the pizza back in the oven. Broil until cheese melts and begins to brown and bubble.

- Remove from the heat. Then cut into 12 slices with a pizza cutter.

- Serve.

Nutrition Facts for 1/12 of the pizza

- Calories 318
- Fiber 1 g
- Protein 21 g
- Fat 23 g
- Carb 8 g

Chapter3
Dinner
Recipes

One Pan Sausage Skillet

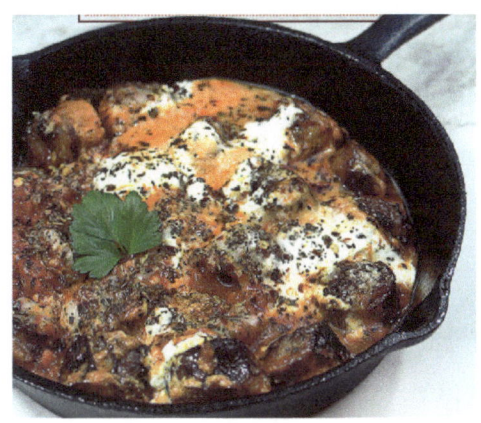

Ingredients for 2 servings

- o   Sausage links – 3

- o   White onion – 1 tablespoon

- o   Mushrooms – 4 oz.

- o   Vodka sauce – ½ cup

- o   Parmesan cheese – ¼ cup

- o   Shredded mozzarella – ¼ cup

- o   Oregano – ½ teaspoon

- o   Basil – ½ teaspoon

- o   Salt – ¼ teaspoon

- o   Red pepper – ¼ teaspoon

Method

1. Preheat the oven to 350F.

2. Heat up a cast iron skillet over medium flame. When the skillet is almost smoking, add your sausage links and cook until they are almost thoroughly cooked.

3. Meanwhile, slice your onion and mushrooms.

4. Take out the sausages when they are almost done. Then add the onions and mushrooms and brown them up a bit.

5. Cut the sausages into rounds (approximately ½ inch in thickness) and then add them back to the skillet. Season your veggie mixture and sausage.

6. Add Parmesan cheese, and pour in your vodka sauce. Stir to combine everything.

7. Place the skillet in the oven and cook for about 15 minutes. Just before the sausage is done, sprinkle mozzarella cheese, so they melt over the top.

8. Cool and serve.

Nutrition Facts Per Serving

- Calories 500
- Fat 38 g
- Protein 30 g
- Carb 4.5 g

Garlicky Shrimp Pasta

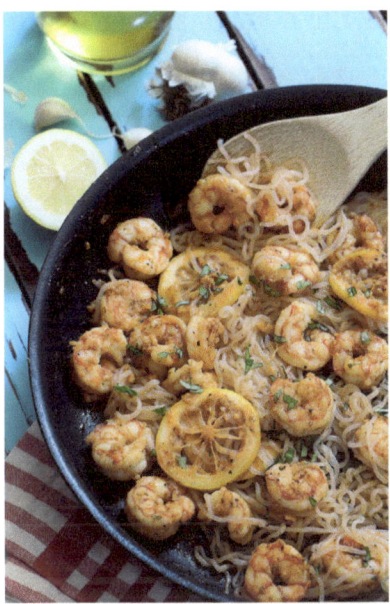

Ingredients for 4 servings

- <u>Miracle Noodle Angel Hair</u> – 2 bags

- Butter – 2 tablespoons

- Olive oil – 2 tablespoons

- Garlic cloves -4, crushed

- Lemon – ½

- Large raw shrimp – 1 lb

- Paprika – ½ teaspoon

- Salt and pepper to taste

- Fresh basil

Method

1. Cook the noodle per package directions.

2. Add the noodle to a dry, hot pan on medium heat. Then dry roast them to remove most of the water. This will make your noodles more flavorful when cooking. Set aside.

3. Add the olive oil and butter in the same pan and let them heat up. Add the garlic cloves to the pan and cook until fragrant, but not brown.

4. Slice the lemons. Add the shrimp and lemon slices to the garlic. Cook until the shrimp are opaque and cooked, about 3 minutes on each side.

5. Add the noodles to the pan and season with paprika, pepper, and salt.

6. Toss everything to coat the noodles in the flavors.

7. Serve with a sprinkle of fresh basil.

Nutrition Facts Per Serving

- Calories 360
- Fat 21 g
- Protein 36 g
- Carb 3.5 g

Salmon with Spinach and Mushrooms

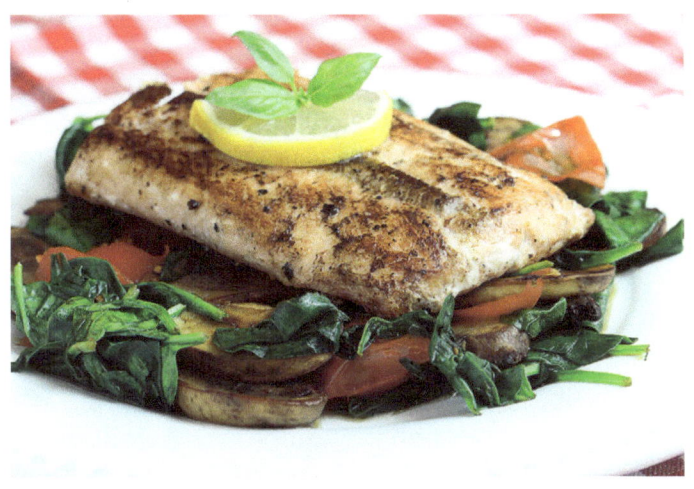

Ingredients for 2 servings

- Olive oil – 1 tablespoon
- Garlic – 2 cloves
- Mushrooms – ½ lb
- Butter – 2 tablespoons
- Campari tomatoes – 2

- Spinach – 2 cups
- Salt and pepper to taste
- Balsamic vinegar – 1 tablespoon
- Olive oil – 1 tablespoon
- Salmon fillets – 2

Method

1. Pat dry your salmon fillets and season both sides with salt and pepper. Keep the fillets in the fridge while you prepare the rest of the ingredients.

2. In a skillet, heat some olive oil over medium heat and slice your mushrooms, tomatoes, and garlic.

3. Cook the mushrooms and garlic in the oil until they shrunk a little. Get them nice and crispy by adding butter to the pan.

4. Add the tomato slices and cook until they denatured a bit.

5. Lastly, add your spinach and cook until it has wilted. Season the mixture with salt and pepper and toss to coat well. Remove from heat and place on a serving plate. Cover with aluminum foil while you cook the fillets.

6. In the same pan, heat another tablespoon olive oil and wait until the oil is very, very hot.

7. Onto the pan, lay the fillets skin side down and sear for 4 to 5 minutes. You might break the fillets, so don't disturb them while they are cooking.

8. Now flip the fillets and cook another 4 to 5 minutes.

9. Then remove the foil from your veggies and drizzle them with balsamic vinegar.

10. Place the salmon on top and garnish with fresh lemon. Serve.

The above salmon meal goes well with garlic cauliflower

Garlic Cauliflower

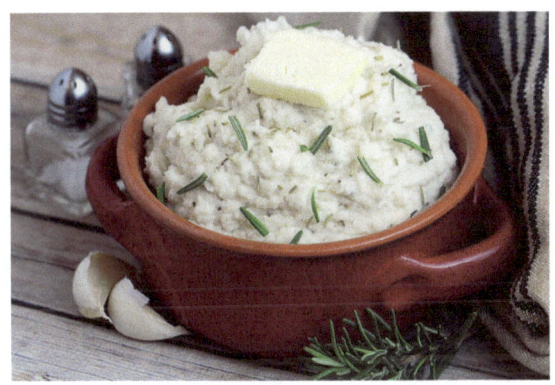

Ingredients for 4 servings

- o   Garlic – 4 cloves

- o   Olive oil – 1 tablespoon

- o   Cauliflower -1/2 head (about 800 grams)

- o   Butter – 4 tablespoons

- o   Rosemary – 2 sprigs or 1 tablespoon

- o   Salt – 1 teaspoon

- o   Pepper – ½ teaspoon

Method

1. With aluminum foil, make a small foil tray to roast your garlic cloves. Place the garlic cloves, drizzle a tablespoon of olive oil and bake in the oven for 10-12 minutes at 400F.

2. Meanwhile, cut the cauliflower into evenly sized florets. Then place the florets into a steam basket over simmering water. Cover with a lid. Steam for 10 minutes, or until a fork pierces through easily.

3. Drain all the water from the pot and place the steamed florets in it. Add the roasted garlic cloves, butter and seasonings.

4. Blend with an immersion blender, until smooth and creamy.

5. Serve.

Nutrition Facts Per Serving

- Calories 200
- Protein 4 g
- Fat 16 g
- Carb 7 g

Chicken Cauliflower Casserole

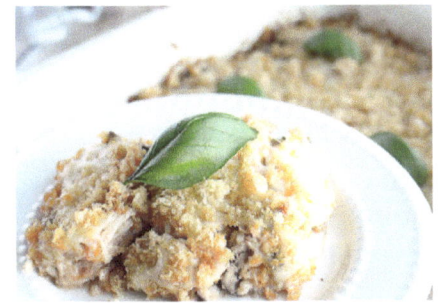

Ingredients for 6 servings

- o   Olive oil – 1 tablespoon
- o   Chicken breast – 20 oz.
- o   Mushrooms – 2.5 oz.
- o   Mayonnaise – ¼ cup
- o   Cauliflower – 2 cups, riced
- o   Heavy cream – ¼ cup
- o   Chicken stock – 1 cup
- o   Low carb vodka sauce – ½ cup
- o   Shredded mozzarella cheese – 1 cup
- o   Pork rinds – 1 oz.
- o   Parmesan cheese – 2 tablespoons
- o   Salt and pepper to taste

- o Oregano

- o Garlicpowder

Method

1. Preheat the oven to 375F.

2. In a pot, cook your cauliflower rice with a cup of boiling chicken broth for 10 to 15 minutes. The liquid from the chicken broth should completely evaporate.

3. Meanwhile, start to cook your chicken breasts. When they are fully cooked, rip the meat apart into bite sized chunks with two forks.

4. To your cooked cauliflower, add ¼ cup of heavy cream and cook for 5 minutes more.

5. Combine the shredded chicken, some sliced mushrooms and ¼ cup of mayonnaise. Mix well.

6. Then add the cauliflower-cream mixture and stir well. Season the mixture with garlic powder, oregano, salt, and pepper.

7. Add the vodka sauce and mix.

8. Place the mixture into a baking dish evenly.

9. Sprinkle with Parmesan cheese, mozzarella cheese and crushed pork rinds for a crunchy finish.

10. Bake until you see the entire dish bubbling, about 20 minutes.

11. Garnish with fresh basil and serve.

Nutrition Facts Per Serving

- Calories 300
- Protein 29 g
- Fat 21 g
- Carb 2.5 g

Chapter 4
Dessert Recipes

Low Carb Brownies

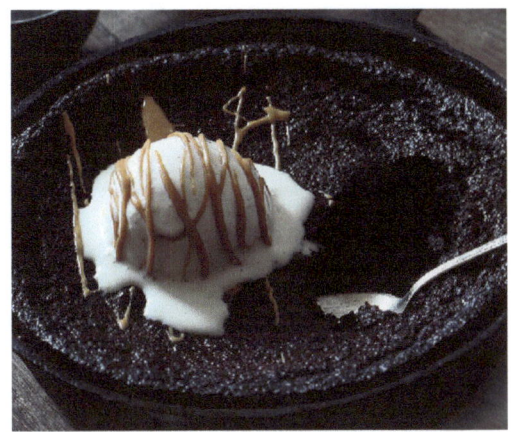

Ingredients for 4 servings

- o   Butter – 6 tablespoons
- o   Erythritol – 1/3 cup
- o   Cocoa powder – 1/3 cup
- o   Egg – 1
- o   Vanilla extract – ½ teaspoon
- o   Salt – 1 pinch
- o   Almond flour – ¼ cup
- o   Baking powder – ½ teaspoon
- o   Walnuts – ¼ cup

Peanut Butter Drizzle

- o   Peanut butter – 1 tablespoon
- o   Butter – 1 tablespoon

Method

1. Preheat the oven to 350F.

2. On a small pan, melt the butter and dissolve erythritol in it. It will take about 5 minutes.

3. Pour the erythritol and butter into a mixing bowl. Then add cocoa powder, vanilla extract, and salt.

4. Add the egg and beat to combine thoroughly.

5. Add the baking powder and almond flour. Add chopped walnuts if desired.

6. Into a 6-inch cast iron skillet, pour your brownie batter.

7. Peanut butter drizzle, in a small pan, melt a tablespoon of peanut butter and a tablespoon of butter. You can add the drizzle after baking or before.

8. Place the skillet into the oven and bake until the top is set, but slightly jiggly, about 30 minutes. Avoid over-baking because brownie will continue to bake while in the skillet.

9. Cool and serve.

Nutrition Facts Per Serving

- Calories 333
- Fat 31.3 g
- Protein 5.8 g
- Carb 3g

Low Carb Cheesecake

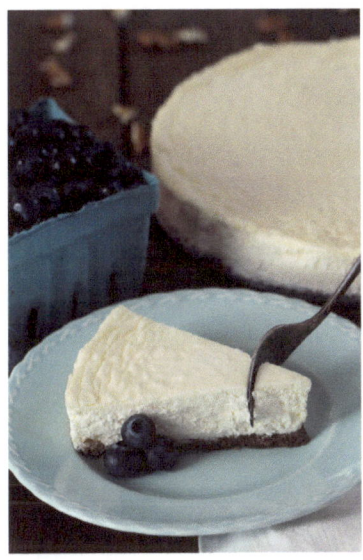

Ingredients for 12 servings

Crust

- o   Almonds – ½ cup

- o   Pecans – ½ cup

- o   Butter – 6 tablespoons (melted)

- o   Protein powder – 1 scoop (31 grams)

- o   Cinnamon – ½ teaspoon

- o   Liquid stevia – 10 drops

- o   Salt – 1 pinch

Cheesecake

- o   Cream cheese – 32 oz.

- ○ Erythritol – 2/3 cup
- ○ Liquid stevia – 20 drops
- ○ Eggs – 4 large
- ○ Vanilla extract – 2 teaspoons
- ○ Fresh lemon juice – 1 teaspoon
- ○ Sour cream – ½ cup
- ○ Pink Himalayan salt – ½ teaspoon

Method

1. Make the crust, on a clean baking sheet, toast the pecans and almonds for 10 minutes in a 325F oven. Toss once so that the nuts are evenly toasted. Don't turn off the oven.

2. In a food processor, add the toasted pecans and almonds with the rest of the crust ingredients and blend until no large chunks of the nuts remain.

3. With a silicone spatula, press the crust into a 9-inch springform pan to make an even, thin layer crust. Bake until the crust has turned golden brown and set about 10 minutes. Let the cooked crust and spring form pan cool before pouring the cheesecake batter.

4. Meanwhile, prepare the cheesecake batter. With an electric hand mixer, beat the stevia, erythritol and cream cheese.

The mixture should be soft and smooth and all the chunks of the cream cheese should be gone.

5. One at a time, add in the eggs, beat until each is incorporated. Then add the lemon juice, vanilla extract, and salt.

6. Add the sour cream and stir until it's combined.

7. By this time the crust should be baked and the spring form pan should be cool. On top of a large sheet of heavy-duty aluminum foil, place the spring form pan and wrap the foil up onto the sides of the spring form pan making sure there are no holes or openings on the bottom. Prepare the spring form for the water bath by placing it into a roasting tray.

8. Now pour the cheesecake batter and with a silicone spatula, smooth out the top. Around the sides of the spring form pan, pour hot water until it's halfway up.

9. Carefully transfer the whole thing to the oven and bake at 325F until the top of the cake is set, but jiggly, about an hour. The cake will continue to cook as it is cooling.

10. When finished baking, turn the oven off. Then crack the door open and leave a wooden spoon wedged in the door. This will allow steady cooling.

11. Leave the cake in the turned off oven for an hour.

12. Then top with your favorite toppings and enjoy.

Nutrition Facts Per Serving

- Calories 415
- Protein 11 g
- Fat 38 g
- Carb 3 g

Almond Coconut Fat Bomb

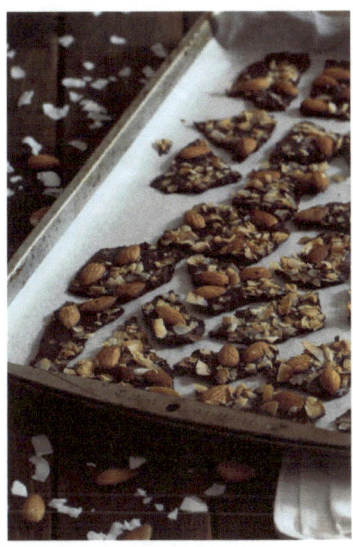

Ingredients for 12 servings

- o   Almonds – ½ cup

- o   Unsweetened flaked coconut – ½ cup

- o   Dark chocolate – 100 grams

- o   Coconut butter – ½ cup

- o   Almond extract – ½ teaspoon

- o   Liquid stevia – 10 drops

- o   Sea salt – ¼ teaspoon

Method

1. Preheat the oven to 350F. Onto a foil-lined baking sheet, spread the coconut and almonds.

2. Place in the oven and toast for about 6 to 8 minutes. Prevent burning by stirring once or twice. Once toasted, set aside to cool.

3. Melt the dark chocolate in a double boiler and once it has melted a bit, stir in the coconut butter. Add in the liquid stevia and almond extract. Mix well and set aside.

4. Line a baking sheet with wax paper or parchment and pour the chocolate mixture in. With a silicone spatula, spread it out evenly.

5. Scatter the toasted coconut flakes and almonds over the top and press gently with your hands so that the nuts and flakes are touching the chocolate. Sprinkle lightly with the sea salt and keep in the refrigerator for at least an hour.

6. When set slice it with a pizza roller.

Nutrition Facts Per Serving

- Calories 173
- Protein 2.8 g
- Fat 15.8 g
- Carb 3.5 g

Double Chocolate Cake

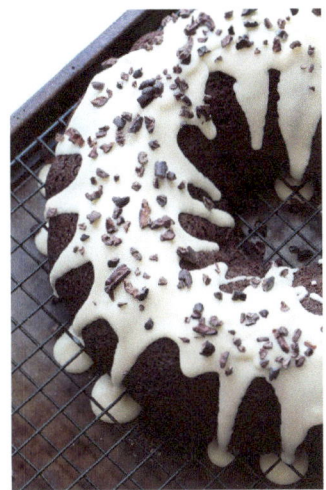

Ingredients for 8 servings

For the Cake

- o   Almond flour – 2 cups

- o   Coconut flour – 2 tablespoons

- o   Erythritol – 1 cup

- o   Baking soda – 1.5 teaspoon

- o   Salt – ½ teaspoon

- o   Butter – 1 cup

- o   Cocoa powder – ½ cup

- o   Water – 1 cup

- o   Eggs – 3 large

- o   Vanilla extract – 2 teaspoons

- o Sour cream – ½ cup

White Chocolate Glaze

- o <u>Organic Cocoa Butter Wafers</u> – 2 oz.

- o Powdered erythritol – 3 tablespoons

- o Vanilla extract – 1 teaspoon

- o Heavy cream – 2 tablespoons

Topping

- o <u>Organic Cocoa Nibs</u> – 20 grams

Method

1. Preheat the oven to 350F.

2. In a bowl, whisk together coconut flour, almond flour, baking soda, erythritol, and salt.

3. Heat together the butter, water and cocoa powder in a small pot on medium heat. Whisk continuously to combine and then remove from the heat.

4. Into the dry mixture, pour in half your chocolate mixture and stir to combine. Once the mixture becomes thick, add the other half and combine.

5. Add in the eggs, one at a time.

6. Then add the vanilla extract and sour cream and stir.

7. Into a greased Bundt cake pan, pour the batter and bake until a wooden skewer stuck into the middle comes out clean, about 40 to 50 minutes.

8. Prepare the white chocolate glaze, while the cake is baking. Start off by melting organic cocoa butter wafers.

9. Now add the powdered erythritol and mix to combine. Add the heavy cream and keep the mixture in the fridge. Stir every 5 minutes.

10. Once the white chocolate is chilled, thick and opaque in color, pulse it in a blender for a few seconds to make it smooth.

11. When the cake is baked, let it cool in the pan for 10-15 minutes. Then cool it completely by placing it onto a cooling rack on a baking sheet.

12. Glaze the cake when the cake is cool to the touch.

13. Sprinkle organic cocoa nibs while the glaze is still wet.

14. Allow the glaze cool and harden. Enjoy.

Nutrition Facts Per Serving

- Calories 520
- Fat 50 g
- Protein 10 g
- Carb5

Conclusion

Lose weight and stay healthy with low carb recipes.